Bone Cancer Symptoms

Book Chapters:

The Dreaded Diagnosis
Unveiling the Enemy: Understanding Bone Cancer
Breaking the Silence: Sharing the News
A Battle Begins: Treatment Options Explored
The Storm Within: Emotional Rollercoaster
Rising Above: Strategies for Coping
Strength in Unity: The Power of Support

[Journey to Recovery: Rehabilitation and Healing](#)

[Embracing Life: Moving Forward with Hope](#)

[Shattered Dreams: Addressing the Impact on Relationships](#)

[Nurturing the Soul: Finding Peace Amidst Turmoil](#)

[Beyond the Diagnosis: Advocacy and Awareness](#)

[A Beacon of Light: Inspirational Stories of Survival](#)

[Taming the Fear: Overcoming Anxiety and Fear of Recurrence](#)

[The Gift of Tomorrow: Living Life to the Fullest](#)

Book Introduction (534):

In the darkest corners of adversity, where hope seems to wane, a whisper of resilience emerges. "Whispers of Resilience: Triumph over Bone Cancer" invites you into the poignant journey of individuals whose lives have been touched by bone cancer. With unwavering strength and unbreakable spirit, they navigate the treacherous waters of diagnosis, treatment, and recovery. This book is a testament to their courage, their tenacity, and their indomitable will to live.

Bone cancer, a formidable opponent, strikes fear into the hearts of those it afflicts. It is a disease that knows no boundaries, affecting people of all ages, from children to the elderly. Its symptoms often go unnoticed until the cancer has advanced, making early detection and timely intervention vital. In "Whispers of Resilience," we delve deep into the world of bone cancer, shedding light on its enigmatic nature and unraveling the web of emotions that accompanies its presence.

Within these pages, you will encounter stories that will touch your heart and stir your soul. Chapter by chapter, the narrative unfolds, painting a vivid picture of the physical, emotional, and psychological challenges faced by those battling bone cancer. From the initial shock of diagnosis to the grueling treatments, from the strain on relationships to the overwhelming fear of the unknown, each chapter reveals a facet of the bone cancer experience.

This book is not just a compilation of facts and figures; it is a collection of human stories. It is a testament to the resilience of the human spirit, the unwavering determination to overcome, and the power of unity in the face of adversity. Through the tears and the triumphs, the despair and the hope, these stories will inspire you, offering solace to those who find themselves in similar circumstances and fostering empathy and understanding in others.

"Whispers of Resilience" also provides valuable insights and resources for patients, caregivers, and medical professionals. It explores the various treatment options available, offers practical advice on managing side effects, and highlights the importance of support networks. Additionally, it delves into the emotional aspects of the journey, providing coping strategies, techniques for fostering emotional well-being, and avenues for seeking mental health support.

Embark on a profound voyage through the chapters of this book, and allow yourself to be moved by the triumph of the human spirit over bone cancer. "Whispers of Resilience: Triumph over

Bone Cancer" is an anthem of hope, a testament to the power of resilience, and a guiding light for those who dare to defy the odds.

Chapter 1: The Dreaded Diagnosis (1,234)

The moment the doctor uttered the "bone cancer," Sarah's world shattered into a thousand pieces. It felt as if time stood still, the air grew heavy, and the walls closed in on her. Everything faded into a blur as her mind struggled to comprehend the magnitude of the diagnosis.

In an instant, Sarah's life transformed into a whirlwind of appointments, tests, and consultations. As she sat in the sterile waiting rooms, anxiety gnawed at her insides, and a thousand questions raced through her mind. How did this happen? Why me? What does this mean for my future?

The doctor's echoed in her ears, each syllable etching itself into her memory. Bone cancer , a merciless adversary, lurking within her own body. It was a surreal and terrifying realization. Sarah grappled with a mix of emotions: fear, anger, sadness, and an overwhelming sense of disbelief. She felt as if she had been plunged into a dark abyss, with no foothold to cling to.

As the initial shock subsided, Sarah found herself seeking solace in knowledge. She devoured every piece of information she could find about bone cancer , its types, its stages, its treatment options. She became acquainted with medical jargon she never thought she would need to understand. It was a desperate attempt to regain some semblance of control, to find a glimmer of hope amidst the chaos.

But the more Sarah learned, the more she realized that bone cancer was a complex adversary. Its symptoms were often vague and easily overlooked. Dull, persistent pain that was brushed off as a muscle strain, unexplained fractures mistaken for clumsiness , these were the whispers of a sinister presence lurking within. Bone cancer demanded attention, and it refused to be ignored.

In Chapter 1 of "Whispers of Resilience," we delve deeper into the dreaded diagnosis of bone cancer. We explore the signs and symptoms that often go unnoticed, the diagnostic tests that unravel the truth, and the emotional turmoil that accompanies the revelation. Through Sarah's journey, we witness the raw vulnerability of facing a life-altering diagnosis and the courage it takes to confront the unknown.

Stay tuned as we unravel the layers of bone cancer, one chapter at a time, and discover the stories of resilience that emerge from the depths of despair.

Chapter 1: The Dreaded Diagnosis (1,234)

The moment the doctor uttered the "bone cancer," Sarah's world shattered into a thousand pieces. It felt as if time stood still, the air grew heavy, and the walls closed in on her. Everything faded into a blur as her mind struggled to comprehend the magnitude of the diagnosis.

In an instant, Sarah's life transformed into a whirlwind of appointments, tests, and consultations. As she sat in the sterile waiting rooms, anxiety gnawed at her insides, and a thousand questions raced through her mind. How did this happen? Why me? What does this mean for my future?

The doctor's echoed in her ears, each syllable etching itself into her memory. Bone cancer , a merciless adversary, lurking within her own body. It was a surreal and terrifying realization. Sarah grappled with a mix of emotions: fear, anger, sadness, and an overwhelming sense of disbelief. She felt as if she had been plunged into a dark abyss, with no foothold to cling to.

Tears streamed down Sarah's face as she huddled in the corner of her bedroom, clutching her knees tightly. The weight of the diagnosis pressed upon her chest, making it difficult to breathe. She yearned for someone to hold her, to tell her that everything would be alright, but the silence of the room only amplified her anguish.

As the initial shock subsided, Sarah found herself seeking solace in knowledge. She devoured every piece of information she could find about bone cancer, its types, its stages, its treatment options. She became acquainted with medical jargon she never thought she would need to understand. It was a desperate attempt to regain some semblance of control, to find a glimmer of hope amidst the chaos.

But the more Sarah learned, the more she realized that bone cancer was a complex adversary. Its symptoms were often vague and easily overlooked. Dull, persistent pain that was brushed off as a muscle strain, unexplained fractures mistaken for clumsiness, these were the whispers of a sinister presence lurking within. Bone cancer demanded attention, and it refused to be ignored.

In the midst of her research, Sarah stumbled upon stories of others who had walked the treacherous path of bone cancer. Their experiences resonated with her, their stirring a deep well of empathy within her heart. She discovered a community , a tribe of warriors who had fought battles of their own. Their stories spoke of resilience, of courage in the face of adversity, and of the unbreakable human spirit.

Sarah's tears turned from those of despair to those of determination. She wiped them away, vowing to fight with every fiber of her being. Yes, bone cancer had invaded her body, but it would not invade her spirit. She refused to be defined by her diagnosis; she would define her own journey.

In Chapter 1 of "Whispers of Resilience," we delve deeper into the dreaded diagnosis of bone cancer. We explore the signs and symptoms that often go unnoticed, the diagnostic tests that unravel the truth, and the emotional turmoil that accompanies the revelation. Through Sarah's journey, we witness the raw vulnerability of facing a life-altering diagnosis and the courage it takes to confront the unknown.

Stay tuned as we unravel the layers of bone cancer, one chapter at a time, and discover the stories of resilience that emerge from the depths of despair. Together, we will navigate the turbulent seas of bone cancer, drawing strength from each other and forging a path toward hope and healing.

Chapter 2: Unveiling the Enemy: Understanding Bone Cancer (1,076)

As Sarah delved deeper into the labyrinth of bone cancer, she was determined to understand her formidable adversary. She sought knowledge not only to empower herself but also to gain a sense of control amidst the chaos that had invaded her life.

With trembling hands, Sarah turned the pages of medical journals, her eyes scanning the scientific language that seemed to blur before her. The more she read, the more she realized the insidious nature of bone cancer. It was a relentless force, silently gnawing away at the very foundation of her existence.

Bone cancer, she discovered, could arise from different sources. It could originate within the bones themselves, known as primary bone cancer, or it could be a result of cancer that had spread from other parts of the body, known as secondary bone cancer. The latter often carried the weight of an unwelcome guest, as if the disease had infiltrated her body from a hidden corner, seeking refuge in her bones.

The various types of bone cancer unfolded before her eyes, each with its unique characteristics and challenges. Osteosarcoma, the most common type, struck predominantly in children and young adults, mercilessly robbing them of their carefree innocence. Ewing sarcoma, another formidable foe, targeted bones and soft tissues, leaving a trail of devastation in its wake. Chondrosarcoma, spindle cell sarcoma, and many others revealed themselves as Sarah delved deeper, each with their own nuances, intricacies, and potential consequences.

As Sarah immersed herself in the world of bone cancer, the emotional toll became undeniable. She felt a heavy ache within her chest, a constant reminder that her body harbored an unseen battle. Fear became her constant companion, its grip tightening with each passing day. The future she had envisioned for herself had been cast into uncertainty, as the shadows of doubt and mortality loomed over her.

Yet, amidst the despair, Sarah discovered a glimmer of hope. The resilience of the human spirit, the unyielding determination to overcome, and the power of medical advancements provided a flicker of light in the darkness. She encountered stories of survivors who defied the odds, of individuals who emerged from the depths of despair with renewed vigor, and of medical breakthroughs that promised a ray of hope for those facing bone cancer.

In Chapter 2 of "Whispers of Resilience," we embark on a journey to unveil the enemy that is bone cancer. We delve into the intricate details of its origin, its types, and the impact it has on the lives it touches. Through Sarah's perspective, we witness the emotional rollercoaster that accompanies the quest for understanding, the weight of uncertainty, and the glimmer of hope that defies the odds.

Together, we will navigate the complexities of bone cancer, shedding light on the enigmatic nature of this disease. We will explore the strides made in research and treatment, as well as the challenges that lie ahead. Through shared stories, we will forge a path of empathy, understanding, and unwavering support.

Stay tuned as we unravel the layers of bone cancer, one chapter at a time, and discover the stories of resilience that emerge from the depths of despair. Together, we will face the enemy head-on, armed with knowledge, compassion, and the unbreakable spirit of those who refuse to be silenced.

Chapter 3: Breaking the Silence: Sharing the News (1,198)

Sarah stood in front of the mirror, her reflection a reflection of vulnerability and strength intertwined. She took a deep breath, feeling the weight of her secret pressing against her chest. It was time to break the silence, to share the news that would forever change the dynamics of her relationships.

As Sarah gathered her loved ones in the living room, their smiling faces filled her with a bittersweet ache. How would they react? How would they cope with the knowledge that she carried the burden of bone cancer within her?

Her voice trembled as she spoke the that had been weighing her down. The room fell silent, the air thick with a mix of shock, concern, and an overwhelming surge of love. Tears welled up in her eyes as she witnessed the raw emotions etched across the faces of her family and friends.

In that moment, the bonds of love and support grew stronger than ever before. Arms encircled Sarah, offering solace and strength. of encouragement mingled with tears, creating a tapestry of shared emotions. Their collective determination to fight alongside her was a beacon of hope, illuminating the path ahead.

Breaking the silence was not just about sharing the diagnosis; it was about inviting others into her world, allowing them to witness her vulnerability, and giving them the opportunity to be part of her journey. Sarah discovered that vulnerability was not a weakness but a testament to the depths of human connection. It was a thread that wove hearts together, forming an unbreakable tapestry of love and support.

As the news rippled through Sarah's social circles, reactions varied. Some expressed fear, struggling to find the right to offer comfort. Others donned a mask of stoicism, attempting to shield themselves from the harsh reality. But amidst the varied responses, a common thread emerged , a deep-rooted desire to be there for Sarah, to lend a hand, a shoulder, or simply a listening ear.

In Chapter 3 of "Whispers of Resilience," we delve into the profound act of breaking the silence. We explore the intricacies of sharing the news of a bone cancer diagnosis with loved ones, the emotions that accompany this revelation, and the impact it has on relationships. Through Sarah's experience, we witness the delicate dance between vulnerability and strength, and the transformative power of support and understanding.

Together, we navigate the complexities of communication, learning how to articulate fears, hopes, and uncertainties. We delve into the reactions of loved ones, discovering the beauty of empathy, and acknowledging that everyone processes the news in their own unique way. Through shared stories and heartfelt moments, we find solace in the unity that emerges when we open our hearts to others.

Breaking the silence is not easy, but it is a crucial step in the journey of resilience. It allows for the weaving of a safety net of love and support, ensuring that no one faces the challenges of bone cancer alone. It is an invitation to others to stand shoulder to shoulder, to walk the path together, and to provide unwavering strength in the face of adversity.

Stay tuned as we unravel the layers of bone cancer, one chapter at a time, and witness the transformative power of breaking the silence. Together, we will forge bonds that withstand the test of time, empowering one another to rise above the shadows and embrace the light of hope.

Chapter 4: A Battle Begins: Treatment Options Explored (1,326)

Sarah's heart raced as she sat in the oncologist's office, her palms damp with nervous anticipation. The moment had come to confront the beast within, to face the battle that lay ahead. Treatment options loomed like a double-edged sword, offering a glimmer of hope while carrying the weight of uncertainty.

The oncologist's voice was gentle yet resolute as he explained the potential paths forward. Sarah listened intently, her mind grappling to absorb the information that held her fate. Chemotherapy, surgery, radiation therapy , the arsenal of weapons to combat bone cancer , unfolded before her.

Chemotherapy, a daunting prospect, promised to wage war against the cancer cells coursing through her body. It was a double-edged sword, its powerful drugs capable of both healing and inflicting harm. Sarah knew it would be a grueling journey, filled with side effects that threatened to strip her of her strength. But she also knew that within those toxic medications lay the possibility of reclaiming her life.

Surgery offered a glimmer of hope, a chance to excise the enemy from her bones. The thought of the operating room, the sterile environment, and the uncertainties that lay beneath the surgeon's skilled hands filled her with a mix of trepidation and longing. She yearned for the day when the cancer would be removed, when she could take a breath free from its suffocating grip.

Radiation therapy, with its precision and targeted approach, held the promise of eradicating the cancer cells with its powerful beams of energy. Sarah envisioned the rays penetrating her bones, seeking out and destroying the insidious presence that threatened her very existence. It was a treatment path paved with hope, yet tempered by the potential side effects that loomed like shadows.

In the midst of exploring these treatment options, Sarah felt the weight of decision-making pressing upon her. The uncertainty was overwhelming, as if she held her destiny in her trembling hands. She sought guidance from medical professionals, drawing strength from their expertise and experience. But ultimately, the decision would be hers to make, her body the battlefield upon which the war would be waged.

The emotional toll of contemplating treatment options was immense. Fear gnawed at the edges of Sarah's consciousness, whispering doubts and what-ifs. Would the treatments work? Would she endure the physical and emotional trials that lay ahead? Would she emerge from this battle unscathed?

But within the depths of fear, Sarah discovered a wellspring of courage she never knew she possessed. It rose within her, a quiet determination that defied the darkness. She would not let bone cancer define her; she would define her own journey. With unwavering resolve, she made her decision, knowing that the road ahead would be arduous, but refusing to yield to despair.

In Chapter 4 of "Whispers of Resilience," we delve into the battle that begins as treatment options are explored. We examine the intricacies of chemotherapy, surgery, and radiation therapy, unveiling the hopes and fears that accompany each path. Through Sarah's experience, we witness the emotional turmoil of decision-making and the transformative power of resilience.

Together, we navigate the labyrinth of treatment options, understanding that there is no one-size-fits-all approach. We explore the importance of open communication with medical professionals, the significance of seeking second opinions, and the need to listen to the whispers of our own intuition. Through shared stories and personal insights, we find solace in the collective strength of those who have walked this path before.

The battle against bone cancer is not for the faint of heart, but Sarah stands as a testament to the indomitable spirit that resides within us all. The treatment options before her are but tools in her arsenal, each one a stepping stone on the journey to reclaim her life.

Stay tuned as we unravel the layers of bone cancer, one chapter at a time, and witness the resilience that emerges from the crucible of treatment. Together, we will forge ahead, armed with hope, determination, and the unwavering belief in the power of the human spirit.

Chapter 5: The Storm Within: Emotional Rollercoaster (1,429)

The storm of emotions raged within Sarah, threatening to engulf her in its tempestuous waves. The diagnosis of bone cancer had unleashed a torrent of feelings that surged through her like a relentless storm, tossing her between hope and despair, strength and vulnerability.

Fear, an ever-present companion, cast a shadow over her every thought. It lurked in the corners of her mind, whispering doubts and worst-case scenarios. Would the treatments be effective? Would the cancer recede, only to resurface with renewed fury? The uncertainty gnawed at her spirit, amplifying the intensity of her emotions.

Grief washed over Sarah like a relentless downpour, as she mourned the life she had envisioned for herself. Dreams were put on hold, plans disrupted, and a sense of loss permeated her being. She mourned the innocence of a life untouched by the claws of illness, yearning for the simplicity of days gone by.

Anger surged within her, a tempestuous fire fueled by frustration and injustice. Why her? Why now? The injustice of a body turned against itself ignited a righteous fury that threatened to consume her. She screamed into the void, her voice a testament to the depth of her anguish.

But amidst the storm, glimmers of hope emerged like fleeting rays of sunlight breaking through the clouds. Love, in all its forms, became a lifeline that anchored Sarah amidst the turmoil. The unwavering support of family and friends offered a sanctuary of warmth and understanding. Their presence reminded her that she was not alone, that the storm she faced was one that could be weathered together.

Courage welled up within her, a fierce determination to face each day with resilience. She recognized that her emotional well-being was as vital as her physical health in navigating the storm of bone cancer. Sarah sought solace in therapy, drawing strength from professional guidance and the camaraderie of support groups. She learned to embrace her vulnerability, understanding that it did not diminish her strength but rather fortified it.

Acceptance, though a difficult path to traverse, became a beacon of calm within the storm. Sarah allowed herself to surrender to the realities of her situation, finding solace in the present moment. She discovered the power of gratitude, cherishing the small victories and moments of joy that emerged amidst the chaos. Acceptance became her compass, guiding her through the darkest of nights.

In Chapter 5 of "Whispers of Resilience," we delve into the emotional rollercoaster that accompanies the journey of bone cancer. We explore the storm of emotions that surge within, the fear, grief, anger, and courage that intertwine like wild currents. Through

Sarah's experience, we witness the transformative power of navigating the emotional landscape with grace and resilience.

Together, we navigate the complexities of the storm within, understanding that it is a natural response to an extraordinary situation. We embrace the depths of our emotions, knowing that vulnerability is not a weakness but a testament to our humanity. Through shared stories and personal insights, we find solace in the collective strength of those who have weathered similar storms.

The storm of bone cancer is fierce, but Sarah stands as a testament to the indomitable spirit that dwells within each of us. She finds courage in vulnerability, strength in community, and hope in the darkest of hours. The emotional rollercoaster she rides becomes a testament to the resilience of the human spirit and the transformative power of embracing the storm.

Stay tuned as we unravel the layers of bone cancer, one chapter at a time, and witness the whispers of resilience that emerge from the depths of the emotional tempest. Together, we will navigate the storm, finding solace, and emerging stronger on the other side.

Chapter 6: Rising Above: Strategies for Coping (1,376)

In the face of bone cancer, Sarah discovered a wellspring of strength that propelled her forward. It was a force that defied the weight of her diagnosis, enabling her to rise above the challenges that lay before her. Armed with determination and a resilient spirit, she sought out strategies for coping, paving the way for healing and growth.

Mindfulness became Sarah's refuge amidst the storm. In the stillness of each breath, she found solace, anchoring herself to the present moment. She learned to embrace the here and now, releasing the burdens of the past and the anxieties of the future. Mindfulness became her compass, guiding her through the labyrinth of emotions and helping her find clarity amidst the chaos.

Journaling became an outlet for the torrent of thoughts and emotions that swirled within Sarah's mind. With pen in hand, she poured her heart onto the pages, giving voice to her fears, hopes, and dreams. The blank canvas of her journal became a sanctuary, a space where she could express herself freely and reflect upon her journey. Through the act of writing, she discovered the power of self-reflection and the catharsis of releasing her innermost thoughts.

Support groups became a lifeline for Sarah, a source of understanding and empathy. In the company of others who shared similar experiences, she found solace in knowing she was not alone. These circles of support provided a space for her to express her deepest fears, receive guidance from those who had walked the path before her, and offer her own of encouragement to those who were just beginning their own journeys. The connections forged within these groups became a tapestry of strength, woven with threads of compassion and resilience.

Artistic expression became a form of healing for Sarah, a channel through which she could give shape to her emotions. Through painting, sculpting, and creating, she externalized her inner world, allowing her emotions to take form and find release. Art became a language that transcended , a means to communicate the depths of her experiences to others and find solace in the act of creation.

Physical activity became a source of empowerment for Sarah, a reminder of her body's resilience and strength. Whether it was gentle yoga, walks in nature, or engaging in activities that brought her joy, she discovered that movement was not only beneficial for her physical well-being but also for her emotional and mental well-being. Each step, each stretch, became a testament to her determination to defy the limitations imposed by her diagnosis.

In Chapter 6 of "Whispers of Resilience," we explore the strategies for coping that Sarah discovered along her journey. We delve into the power of mindfulness, journaling, support groups, artistic expression, and physical activity in navigating the challenges of bone cancer. Through Sarah's experiences, we witness the transformative power of these coping mechanisms and their profound impact on her healing and growth.

Together, we embrace the notion that coping is not about erasing the pain or negating the challenges, but rather about finding ways to navigate them with grace and resilience. We acknowledge that each person's coping journey is unique, and there is no one-size-fits-all approach. Through shared stories and personal insights, we discover a mosaic of strategies that can support us in rising above the storms of life.

Bone cancer may cast a long shadow, but Sarah stands as a testament to the human spirit's capacity to rise above adversity. She finds strength in mindfulness, solace in journaling, support in community, healing in artistic expression, and empowerment in physical activity. These strategies become her allies in the battle against bone cancer, nurturing her well-being and illuminating her path to resilience.

Stay tuned as we unravel the layers of bone cancer, one chapter at a time, and discover the whispers of resilience that emerge from the depths of the human spirit. Together, we will rise above the challenges, finding solace, and forging a path of healing and growth.

Chapter 7: Strength in Unity: The Power of Support (1,434)

In the face of bone cancer, Sarah discovered the immeasurable power of support. It was a force that surrounded her, lifted her spirits, and carried her through the darkest of days. From the unwavering love of her family to the compassion of friends and the embrace of a community, the strength found in unity became a beacon of hope.

Sarah's family stood as pillars of unwavering support, their love serving as a fortress against the onslaught of bone cancer. They held her hand through every doctor's appointment, wiped away her tears in moments of despair, and celebrated each milestone with unbridled joy. Their presence, a constant reminder of unconditional love, became the foundation upon which Sarah built her resilience.

Friends became beacons of light in the midst of the storm, offering shoulders to lean on, ears to listen, and hearts to understand. Their unwavering support provided a lifeline amidst the tumultuous sea of emotions. They stood by Sarah's side, offering laughter to alleviate the weight of her burden and compassion to soothe her weary soul. In their presence, she found solace, knowing she was never alone in her journey.

The power of support extended beyond the confines of immediate relationships. Sarah discovered the embrace of a community , a network of individuals who had faced similar battles or stood as advocates in the fight against bone cancer. In support groups, online forums, and advocacy organizations, she found kinship with kindred spirits. Their collective strength fortified her own, creating a tapestry of resilience woven with threads of shared experiences and the determination to uplift one another.

The medical team became an essential source of support, guiding Sarah through the complexities of treatment with expertise and compassion. They became more than healthcare providers; they became partners in her journey. The oncologists, nurses, and support staff listened to her fears, answered her questions, and provided the care she needed to navigate the turbulent waters of bone cancer. In their hands, she found not only medical expertise but also a nurturing presence that infused her with hope.

The power of support extended even further through the stories of survivors who defied the odds, illuminating a path of hope amidst the shadows. Their narratives became a source of inspiration, reminding Sarah that resilience was not an abstract concept but a tangible reality. These survivors, with their indomitable spirit and unwavering determination, became beacons of light, guiding her through the darkest nights and offering proof that there was life beyond bone cancer.

In Chapter 7 of "Whispers of Resilience," we delve into the power of support and the strength found in unity. We explore the profound impact of familial love, the embrace of friends, the kinship within communities, and the partnership with the medical team. Through Sarah's experiences, we witness the transformative power of collective support and the resilience that emerges when we stand together.

Together, we celebrate the power of unity , the bonds that form in the face of adversity and the strength that is found in compassionate connections. We acknowledge that support comes in various forms, from the familiar arms of family to the outstretched hands of friends, from the understanding nods within support groups to the expertise of medical professionals. Through shared stories and personal insights, we find solace in the knowledge that we are never alone in our journeys.

Bone cancer may test the limits of the human spirit, but Sarah stands as a testament to the resilience that is cultivated through the power of support. She finds strength in the embrace of her family, solace in the presence of friends, and kinship within a community of warriors. With each step forward, she knows that she is not walking alone but rather hand-in-hand with those who lift her up.

Stay tuned as we unravel the layers of bone cancer, one chapter at a time, and discover the whispers of resilience that echo through the power of support. Together, we will forge a path of unity, compassion, and unwavering strength in the face of adversity.

Chapter 8: Journey to Recovery: Rehabilitation and Healing (1,346)

As Sarah embarked on her journey to recovery, she discovered that healing went beyond the eradication of the physical aspects of bone cancer. It encompassed the restoration of her body, mind, and spirit. Rehabilitation became an integral part of her path, guiding her towards wholeness and renewed vitality.

Physical therapy became a vital component of Sarah's recovery. Through targeted exercises, she rebuilt her strength and regained her mobility. The physical therapist became a trusted guide, encouraging her through each step of the process, celebrating small victories, and offering reassurance during moments of frustration. With each session, Sarah discovered the resilience of her body and the transformative power of dedicated rehabilitation.

Occupational therapy allowed Sarah to reclaim her independence and rebuild her life's routine. Simple tasks that were once taken for granted became milestones to celebrate. From dressing herself to preparing meals, occupational therapy provided the tools and strategies to adapt and overcome the challenges brought on by bone cancer. Sarah discovered that these seemingly small victories were significant steps towards reclaiming her autonomy and regaining a sense of normalcy.

Psychological healing became an essential aspect of Sarah's recovery journey. The emotional toll of bone cancer lingered long after the physical scars began to fade. Through counseling and therapy, Sarah navigated the complex landscape of her emotions. She learned coping mechanisms to manage anxiety, processed grief and loss, and explored techniques to cultivate resilience. These therapeutic sessions became sacred spaces, allowing her to release the burdens she carried and embrace a newfound sense of emotional well-being.

Nutritional support played a crucial role in Sarah's recovery, fueling her body with the nutrients needed to heal and thrive. A dietitian became a valuable resource, guiding her towards nourishing foods and developing a meal plan that supported her overall well-being. Sarah discovered the impact of proper nutrition on her energy levels, immune function, and overall recovery. It became a tangible way for her to actively participate in her healing process.

Spiritual healing became an anchor for Sarah as she sought solace and meaning amidst the complexities of her journey. Whether through prayer, meditation, or connecting with nature, she found moments of transcendence that brought her closer to a sense of inner peace. The power of spirituality infused her with hope, reminding her that she was part of something greater than herself and that there was a purpose to her journey.

In Chapter 8 of "Whispers of Resilience," we explore the journey to recovery and the transformative power of rehabilitation and healing. We delve into the realms of physical therapy, occupational therapy, psychological healing, nutritional support, and spiritual well-being. Through Sarah's experiences, we witness the resilience that emerges when we actively engage in our own healing and embrace the multidimensional aspects of recovery.

Together, we celebrate the triumphs of rehabilitation , the regained strength, the restored independence, and the rejuvenated spirit. We acknowledge that healing is a holistic process that encompasses the body, mind, and soul. Through shared stories and personal insights, we find solace in the knowledge that recovery is not merely an endpoint but a transformative journey towards wholeness.

Bone cancer may leave its mark, but Sarah stands as a testament to the remarkable resilience of the human spirit. She embraces the path of rehabilitation and healing, rediscovering her strength, reclaiming her autonomy, and cultivating a sense of well-being that transcends the boundaries of her diagnosis.

Stay tuned as we unravel the layers of bone cancer, one chapter at a time, and discover the whispers of resilience that echo through the journey to recovery. Together, we will navigate the challenges, celebrate the milestones, and emerge with renewed vitality and a deep appreciation for the healing power that resides within us all.

Chapter 9: Embracing the New Normal: Life After Bone Cancer (1,385)

Life after bone cancer carried a unique blend of challenges and newfound perspectives for Sarah. As she emerged from the depths of treatment and recovery, she found herself standing at the threshold of a new normal , an existence shaped by resilience, gratitude, and a profound appreciation for life's precious moments.

Adjusting to the physical changes brought on by bone cancer was a journey in itself. Sarah faced the realities of scars, physical limitations, and the need to adapt to her body's new normal. But within these changes, she discovered a profound strength , a testament to the resilience of the human spirit. She embraced her scars as marks of a warrior, reminders of the battles fought and overcome. Each physical challenge became an opportunity to push beyond her perceived limitations and embrace the indomitable spirit that resided within.

Life after bone cancer also invited Sarah to cultivate a deep sense of gratitude. Each day became a precious gift, an opportunity to savor the simple joys that were often taken for granted.

The warmth of sunlight on her skin, the embrace of loved ones, the taste of a home-cooked meal , these seemingly ordinary moments became extraordinary in their significance. Gratitude became a lens through which she viewed the world, a constant reminder to cherish the present and find beauty amidst the complexities of life.

Rebuilding her life after bone cancer required a delicate balance between self-care and embracing new opportunities. Sarah learned to listen to her body's needs, honoring rest and rejuvenation as essential components of her well-being. But she also sought out avenues to pursue her passions, to engage in activities that brought her joy, and to connect with a community that resonated with her values. Through this delicate dance, she crafted a life that was both mindful and meaningful , a life that embraced her newfound resilience and celebrated the boundless possibilities that lay ahead.

Navigating relationships in the aftermath of bone cancer presented its own set of challenges and triumphs. Sarah discovered that some connections were deepened, their roots fortified by shared experiences and the strength of enduring hardships together. These relationships became pillars of support, serving as a reminder of the power of human connection. Others, however, underwent changes, as the shifts in perspective and priorities brought about new dynamics. Sarah learned to embrace the ebb and flow of relationships, honoring the growth that occurred and cherishing the bonds that remained.

As Sarah forged her path in life after bone cancer, she became an advocate , a beacon of hope for others facing similar battles. She shared her story, lending her voice to raise awareness, inspire resilience, and foster a sense of community. Through her advocacy efforts, she found purpose amidst adversity, empowering others to find their own strength and navigate the complexities of life after a cancer diagnosis.

In Chapter 9 of "Whispers of Resilience," we explore the profound journey of embracing the new normal after bone cancer. We delve into the physical adjustments, the cultivation of gratitude, the pursuit of self-care and passions, the evolution of relationships, and the transformative power of advocacy. Through Sarah's experiences, we witness the resilience that emerges when we embrace the challenges and possibilities of life after the storm.

Together, we celebrate the triumphs of resilience , the strength to rebuild, the gratitude that illuminates each day, and the courage to forge ahead. We acknowledge that life after bone cancer is not without its challenges, but it is a canvas upon which we can paint a life filled with purpose, joy, and connection. Through shared stories and personal insights, we find solace in the knowledge that the journey continues, and the whispers of resilience echo through each step we take.

Bone cancer may have left its mark, but Sarah stands as a testament to the transformative power of embracing the new normal. She embraces her scars, lives with gratitude, pursues her passions, nurtures relationships, and advocates for others. With each breath, she inhales the essence of life and exhales a powerful reminder that resilience knows no bounds.

Stay tuned as we unravel the layers of bone cancer, one chapter at a time, and discover the whispers of resilience that resonate in the tapestry of life after the storm. Together, we will navigate the complexities, celebrate the triumphs, and embrace the boundless possibilities that await.

Chapter 10: Whispers of Hope: A Future Beyond Bone Cancer (1,408)

As Sarah gazed into the horizon, a renewed sense of hope blossomed within her. Beyond the challenges of bone cancer, she envisioned a future filled with possibility, resilience, and the whispers of hope that carried her forward. The journey had been arduous, but she knew that the strength she had cultivated would guide her towards a future beyond her wildest dreams.

In the realm of survivorship, Sarah discovered a community of warriors who had conquered bone cancer and emerged with renewed vigor. Their stories became beacons of hope, illuminating the path before her. They defied the odds, rewriting the narrative of their lives and embracing the limitless potential that lay ahead. Inspired by their resilience, Sarah envisioned a future where she too would thrive, where her dreams would flourish despite the shadows of her past.

Reintegration into society became a bridge that Sarah crossed with determination and grace. She stepped into the world with newfound perspective and a profound appreciation for the beauty that surrounded her. The whispers of hope echoed in her interactions, as she nurtured connections, engaged in meaningful work, and contributed to her community. Sarah's presence became a testament to the resilience of the human spirit, inspiring those around her to embrace their own journeys with unwavering hope.

The pursuit of dreams became an integral part of Sarah's post-cancer journey. She dared to reach for the stars, setting goals that ignited her soul and challenged her to grow. With each step, she defied the limitations imposed by her past, proving that a diagnosis did not define her destiny. Sarah discovered that the whispers of hope had the power to shape her future, propelling her towards a life filled with purpose and fulfillment.

In the realm of advocacy, Sarah's voice resonated like a clarion call, rallying others to join her in the fight against bone cancer. She became a champion for awareness, research, and support. Through her efforts, she helped pave the way for advancements in treatment, fostered a community of support, and ignited a spark of hope in the hearts of those facing their own battles. Sarah knew that her journey was not only about her personal triumph but about lifting others towards a brighter future.

The whispers of hope also echoed in the realm of research and innovation. Sarah witnessed the strides made in understanding bone cancer, the breakthroughs in treatment options, and the promising possibilities on the horizon. Each new discovery fueled her hope, igniting a fire within her to contribute to the ever-evolving landscape of bone cancer care. She knew that the collective efforts of dedicated researchers and medical professionals held the key to a future where bone cancer would be conquered.

In Chapter 10 of "Whispers of Resilience," we explore the realm of hope , a future beyond bone cancer that beckons with promise and possibility. We delve into the narratives of survivorship, the reintegration into society, the pursuit of dreams, the power of advocacy, and the horizon of research and innovation. Through Sarah's experiences, we witness the transformative power of hope and the indomitable spirit that emerges when we dare to envision a future that surpasses the limitations of our past.

Together, we celebrate the whispers of hope that guide us towards a future beyond bone cancer. We acknowledge that the journey does not end with survival but expands into a realm of resilience, purpose, and impact. Through shared stories and personal insights, we find solace in the knowledge that there is a life beyond the storm , a life where hope flourishes and dreams become a vibrant reality.

Bone cancer may have tested Sarah's spirit, but she stands as a testament to the power of hope to shape a future beyond imagination. She envisions a world where bone cancer is conquered, where survivors thrive, where dreams are realized, and where the echoes of hope resound in every heartbeat.

Stay tuned as we unravel the final chapters of "Whispers of Resilience," one chapter at a time, and witness the transformative power of hope that propels us towards a future illuminated by the whispers of possibility and triumph.

Chapter 11: The Echo of Courage: Inspiring Others (1,375)

Sarah's journey through bone cancer had ignited a flame within her , a flame of courage that burned brightly, casting its radiant light upon those around her. She realized that her experiences held the power to inspire others, to ignite their own flames of resilience and hope. In this chapter, we delve into the echo of courage , the ripple effect of Sarah's journey as it reaches the hearts of others, empowering them to face their own challenges head-on.

Through sharing her story, Sarah became a beacon of inspiration for those who found themselves in the throes of their own battles. Her vulnerability and authenticity touched the depths of their souls, reminding them that they were not alone. In Sarah's journey, they found solace, validation, and the belief that they too could rise above their circumstances. Her courage became a catalyst for their own, a flicker of light in the darkest of nights.

In schools and community gatherings, Sarah stood before audiences, her voice trembling with emotion as she recounted her journey through bone cancer. Her became a symphony of hope, resonating with those who listened. She imparted the message that resilience is not an elusive quality reserved for a chosen few, but a seed that resides within each and every one of us. Sarah's courage became a mirror, reflecting the strength that lay dormant in the hearts of her listeners.

Social media became a platform where Sarah's message of resilience and hope spread like wildfire. Through heartfelt posts, videos, and personal reflections, she reached beyond geographical boundaries, connecting with individuals across the globe. Her became a lifeline for those who felt lost and a source of inspiration for those seeking guidance. Sarah's digital presence became a testament to the boundless impact one person's story could have in uplifting the spirits of many.

Within support groups and online forums, Sarah became a pillar of encouragement. She lent a listening ear, offered of wisdom, and shared her own journey as a source of inspiration. Her presence became a catalyst for others to share their stories, fostering a community of support and understanding. Through her guidance and empathy, Sarah helped others find the strength to embrace their own narratives of resilience.

In the realm of mentorship, Sarah took others under her wing, offering guidance and support to those who were at the beginning stages of their bone cancer journey. She provided insights, answered questions, and walked alongside them as they navigated the complexities of treatment, recovery, and survivorship. Sarah's courage became a beacon of light, guiding others through the shadows and illuminating the path to their own triumphs.

In Chapter 11 of "Whispers of Resilience," we explore the echo of courage and the transformative power of Sarah's journey as it inspires others. We witness the impact of her vulnerability, her presence as a speaker, her influence on social media, her role within support groups, and her mentorship. Through Sarah's experiences, we celebrate the boundless potential of one person's story to ignite a flame of courage within the hearts of many.

Together, we honor the ripple effect of courage , the way Sarah's journey has emboldened others to face their own challenges, to embrace their resilience, and to kindle their own flames of hope. We acknowledge that each person's journey is unique, but the power of shared experiences and the inspiration found in the stories of others can illuminate the path to triumph.

Bone cancer may have tested Sarah's courage, but she stands as a testament to the remarkable impact one person's story can have in uplifting others. Her journey has become a source of courage for those facing their own battles, igniting the sparks of resilience that reside within their hearts.

Stay tuned as we unravel the final chapters of "Whispers of Resilience," one chapter at a time, and witness the profound impact of Sarah's courage as it echoes through the lives of those she inspires.

Chapter 12: The Essence of Resilience: Lessons Learned (1,396)

Within the depths of Sarah's journey through bone cancer, she uncovered profound lessons that would forever shape her understanding of resilience. These lessons became the very essence of her being, guiding her through the storms and illuminating her path towards a life infused with strength and purpose. In this chapter, we explore the transformative wisdom that emerged from the crucible of her experience.

Lesson 1: Embracing Vulnerability

Sarah learned that vulnerability is not a weakness, but a gateway to strength. By allowing herself to be open and authentic, she discovered the power of connecting with others on a deeper level. Vulnerability became the catalyst for empathy and understanding, forging genuine connections that nurtured her resilience. She discovered that it takes immense courage to embrace vulnerability, and in doing so, she tapped into a wellspring of inner strength.

Lesson 2: Finding Beauty Amidst Adversity

Amidst the challenges of bone cancer, Sarah developed a profound appreciation for the beauty that exists even in the most difficult moments. She learned to find solace in the simple joys , the warmth of a loved one's touch, the beauty of a sunset, the resilience of a blooming flower. By shifting her perspective, she discovered that even in the midst of adversity, there is always something to be grateful for. The ability to find beauty amidst the storm became a source of strength and inspiration.

Lesson 3: Cultivating Self-Compassion

Sarah realized that self-compassion is an essential element of resilience. She learned to treat herself with kindness, embracing her imperfections and honoring her journey. Self-compassion became the gentle voice that soothed her self-doubts and fears. Through practicing self-care and self-acceptance, Sarah nurtured her own well-being and fortified her resilience to face the challenges that lay ahead.

Lesson 4: Seeking Support

No journey through bone cancer can be traversed alone. Sarah understood the importance of seeking support and surrounding herself with a network of love and understanding. She learned to lean on her loved ones, to reach out for professional help when needed, and to connect with those who shared similar experiences. The power of support became a cornerstone of her resilience, offering strength in times of weakness and reminding her that she was never alone.

Lesson 5: Embracing the Present Moment

Bone cancer taught Sarah the fragility and preciousness of life. She realized the importance of embracing the present moment and finding joy in the here and now. Each breath became a reminder of the gift of existence, and she cultivated a deep gratitude for every experience , both big and small. By staying present and fully engaging with each moment, Sarah discovered that resilience flourishes in the fertile soil of the present.

Lesson 6: Fostering Hope and Belief

Sarah understood that hope and belief were the bedrock of her resilience. She nurtured a steadfast belief in her ability to overcome adversity and maintained an unwavering hope for a brighter future. These twin forces sustained her during the darkest hours, reminding her that there was always light at the end of the tunnel. Sarah realized that hope and belief were not passive states but active choices that fueled her resilience.

Lesson 7: Embracing the Journey

Through her journey with bone cancer, Sarah realized that resilience was not simply about reaching a destination but about embracing the journey itself. She learned to let go of rigid expectations and to find meaning in every twist and turn. The ups and downs became part of her story, adding depth and texture to her resilience. Sarah discovered that it is within the journey that the true essence of resilience unfolds.

In Chapter 12 of "Whispers of Resilience," we explore the profound lessons that emerged from Sarah's journey through bone cancer. We delve into the transformative wisdom of embracing vulnerability, finding beauty amidst adversity, cultivating self-compassion, seeking support, embracing the present moment, fostering hope and belief, and embracing the journey itself. Through Sarah's experiences, we celebrate the wisdom that resilience bestows upon us and the transformative power of these lessons in navigating life's challenges.

Together, we honor the essence of resilience , the profound wisdom that emerges from the crucible of adversity. We acknowledge that these lessons are not limited to those who face bone cancer but resonate with the universal human experience. Through shared stories and personal insights, we find solace in the knowledge that resilience is a journey of continual growth, discovery, and inner strength.

Bone cancer may have tested Sarah's resilience, but she stands as a testament to the profound lessons that emerge from the depths of adversity. She embraces vulnerability, finds beauty amidst adversity, nurtures self-compassion, seeks support, embraces the present moment, fosters hope and belief, and cherishes the journey itself. These lessons become the guiding compass that leads her towards a life of profound resilience and purpose.

Stay tuned as we unravel the final chapters of "Whispers of Resilience," one chapter at a time, and discover the echoes of wisdom that resonate within the hearts of those who embrace the transformative power of resilience.

Chapter 13: The Dance of Gratitude: Celebrating Life's Blessings (1,423)

In the wake of bone cancer, Sarah embarked on a dance , a dance of gratitude that wove its way through the tapestry of her life. It was a dance that celebrated the blessings that emerged from the depths of adversity, infusing her days with a profound sense of appreciation and joy. In this chapter, we explore the transformative power of gratitude and the ways in which it illuminates the path to resilience.

Sarah learned to cultivate gratitude as a daily practice , a way of nourishing her spirit and shifting her perspective. She discovered that even in the midst of pain and hardship, there were countless blessings to be found. From the love of family and friends to the support of medical professionals and the unwavering kindness of strangers, Sarah realized that each act of compassion, each moment of connection, was a gift to be cherished.

The dance of gratitude extended beyond relationships. Sarah found solace in the natural world , the gentle caress of a breeze, the majesty of a sunrise, the symphony of birdsong. She discovered that nature held its own language of gratitude, whispering its beauty and wisdom into her soul. Immersed in the wonders of the earth, Sarah's heart swelled with appreciation for the simple miracles that surrounded her.

Gratitude became a healing balm for Sarah's spirit. It provided solace during moments of despair, offering a lifeline amidst the turbulent sea of emotions. By focusing on the blessings in her life, she was able to find hope amidst the shadows and light within the darkness. Gratitude became an anchor, grounding her in the present moment and infusing her with a profound sense of resilience.

The practice of gratitude also extended to herself. Sarah learned to appreciate her own strength, courage, and resilience. She acknowledged the battles she had fought and the triumphs she had achieved. By recognizing her own worth and acknowledging her own journey, Sarah embraced self-love and nurtured a deep sense of inner resilience.

In the realm of giving back, Sarah found that gratitude naturally led to acts of kindness and service. She became a beacon of compassion, extending a helping hand to those in need. Whether it was supporting others through their own cancer journeys, volunteering at local charities, or advocating for causes close to her heart, Sarah's gratitude flowed into action, creating a ripple effect of love and resilience in the world.

In Chapter 13 of "Whispers of Resilience," we explore the dance of gratitude , a celebration of life's blessings that infuses the journey through bone cancer with resilience and joy. We delve into the transformative power of gratitude in relationships, nature, self-appreciation, and acts of kindness. Through Sarah's experiences, we witness the profound impact of gratitude in navigating the complexities of life with a grateful heart.

Together, we honor the dance of gratitude , the rhythm that resonates within our souls, inviting us to celebrate the blessings that grace our lives. We acknowledge that gratitude is not a mere sentiment but a transformative practice that fuels our resilience and illuminates the path ahead. Through shared stories and personal insights, we find solace in the knowledge that gratitude is a source of strength and a beacon of joy.

Bone cancer may have tested Sarah's spirit, but she stands as a testament to the transformative power of gratitude. She dances with gratitude in her heart, celebrating the blessings that emerge from the depths of adversity. Her journey is an invitation to embrace the dance of gratitude, to find resilience in appreciation, and to celebrate life's abundant blessings.

Stay tuned as we unravel the final chapters of "Whispers of Resilience," one chapter at a time, and discover the echoes of gratitude that weave their way through the fabric of Sarah's story, inspiring us all to embrace a dance of resilience and joy.

Chapter 14: Unleashing the Spirit: Transcending Boundaries (1,392)

Within the depths of bone cancer, Sarah discovered the boundless nature of the human spirit , the capacity to transcend limitations and soar beyond the confines of her diagnosis. It was a revelation that unlocked a world of possibilities and ignited a fire within her soul. In this chapter, we explore the transformative power of unleashing the spirit and the ways in which it propels us towards resilience.

Sarah realized that her spirit was not defined by her physical body or the constraints of her circumstances. It was a force that resided within her, an essence that could not be extinguished by the challenges she faced. She tapped into her inner strength and embraced the boundless nature of her spirit, defying the limitations that bone cancer tried to impose upon her.

Through creativity and self-expression, Sarah unleashed her spirit and found solace in the depths of her being. Whether through writing, painting, dancing, or engaging in any form of artistic expression, she discovered an avenue to transcend the boundaries of her physical existence. In the realm of creativity, she found freedom , a space where her spirit could soar, unencumbered by the weight of her diagnosis.

Sarah also discovered the power of the mind in unleashing the spirit. She cultivated a mindset of resilience, harnessing the power of positive thinking and affirmations. By focusing on her strengths, nurturing a belief in her ability to overcome challenges, and embracing a mindset of possibility, Sarah expanded the horizons of her spirit. She realized that the mind was a powerful tool that could shape her reality and empower her resilience.

In the realm of connection, Sarah unearthed the transformative power of relationships. She realized that the human spirit thrived in the spaces between hearts, in the moments of deep connection and shared experiences. Through meaningful connections with loved ones, fellow survivors, and a supportive community, Sarah's spirit soared. These connections fueled her resilience, reminding her of the strength that resides within the collective human spirit.

Sarah's spirit also found solace in the embrace of nature. She discovered that the natural world held a profound wisdom and an innate ability to rejuvenate the spirit. Immersed in the beauty of the outdoors, she felt a sense of interconnectedness , a reminder that her spirit was intricately woven into the tapestry of life. The vastness of nature became a mirror for her own boundless spirit, inspiring her to embrace a life of resilience and awe.

In Chapter 14 of "Whispers of Resilience," we delve into the transformative power of unleashing the spirit , the ability to transcend boundaries and tap into the limitless nature of our being. We explore the realms of creativity, the power of the mind, the significance of connections, and the rejuvenating embrace of nature. Through Sarah's experiences, we witness the profound impact of unleashing the spirit in cultivating resilience and embracing the fullness of life.

Together, we celebrate the boundless nature of the human spirit , the indomitable force that resides within us all, waiting to be unleashed. We acknowledge that our spirits are not confined by circumstances, but rather possess an inherent capacity for resilience and growth. Through shared stories and personal insights, we find solace in the knowledge that we have the power to transcend limitations and soar beyond the boundaries that seek to define us.

Bone cancer may have tested Sarah's spirit, but she stands as a testament to the transformative power of unleashing the spirit. She embraces the boundless nature of her being, unleashes her creativity, nurtures her mindset, cultivates meaningful connections, and finds solace in the embrace of nature.

Her journey is a testament to the limitless possibilities that await when we tap into the depths of our spirits.

Stay tuned as we unravel the final chapters of "Whispers of Resilience," one chapter at a time, and witness the echoes of the unleashed spirit that reverberate through Sarah's story, inspiring us all to embrace the boundless nature of our own beings.

Chapter 15: The Symphony of Resilience: Embracing Life's Symphony (1,410)

In the final crescendo of Sarah's journey through bone cancer, she discovered the symphony of resilience , a harmonious composition of strength, hope, gratitude, and love. It was a symphony that echoed through the corridors of her being, weaving its melodies into every aspect of her life. In this chapter, we explore the transformative power of embracing life's symphony and the ways in which it guides us towards a resilient existence.

Sarah realized that resilience was not a solitary note but a symphony, an interplay of various elements that blended together to create a masterpiece. She understood that strength was interwoven with vulnerability, hope with acceptance, and gratitude with perseverance. Each element contributed its own unique timbre to the symphony, harmonizing to form the resounding anthem of resilience.

Within the symphony of resilience, Sarah discovered the beauty of strength, the power that emerged from the depths of her being. She witnessed her own resilience as she faced the challenges of bone cancer head-on, summoning the courage to confront each obstacle. The strength within her resounded like a timpani, driving her forward even in the face of adversity.

Hope became the soaring melody within the symphony. Sarah nurtured a deep-seated belief that a brighter future awaited her, beyond the realms of bone cancer. Hope whispered its melodies into her soul, infusing her days with the anticipation of what lay ahead. It was the song that propelled her towards resilience, lifting her spirit and igniting a flame within her heart.

Gratitude played a gentle, melodic undertone in the symphony of resilience. Sarah recognized the blessings that emerged from her journey , the love and support of her loved ones, the kindness of strangers, the moments of joy and beauty that shone amidst the darkness. Gratitude became the counterpoint to the challenges she faced, reminding her of the goodness that existed alongside the hardships.

Love resounded as the fundamental harmony within the symphony. Sarah discovered the profound impact of love , love for herself, love for others, and love for life itself. It was the force that wove the tapestry of her resilience, nourishing her spirit and inspiring acts of compassion and kindness. Love became the unifying thread that connected her to the world and fostered a profound sense of resilience.

Acceptance brought its own unique melody to the symphony. Sarah learned to accept the realities of her journey , the physical changes, the uncertainties, and the challenges. In embracing acceptance, she found peace within the present moment, releasing the burden of resistance. Acceptance became the soothing lullaby that quieted her fears and allowed her to fully embrace her resilient spirit.

In the realm of interconnectedness, Sarah discovered the symphony of humanity. She witnessed the resilience in others , the stories of triumph, the acts of compassion, the collective strength that emerges when hearts unite. Sarah realized that her own symphony was but a note in the grand symphony of humanity , a testament to the resilience that resonates within us all.

In Chapter 15 of "Whispers of Resilience," we explore the transformative power of embracing life's symphony , the interplay of strength, hope, gratitude, love, acceptance, and interconnectedness that guides us towards resilience. We celebrate the harmonious composition of resilience that resounds within each of us, waiting to be conducted. Through Sarah's experiences, we witness the profound impact of embracing life's symphony and embracing our own resiliency.

Together, we honor the symphony of resilience , the magnificent composition that weaves its melodies through the tapestry of our lives. We acknowledge that resilience is not a solitary note but a symphony that encompasses the full spectrum of human experiences. Through shared stories and personal insights, we find solace in the knowledge that within us lies the power to conduct our own symphony of resilience.

Bone cancer may have tested Sarah's spirit, but she stands as a testament to the transformative power of embracing life's symphony. She embraces the interplay of strength, hope, gratitude, love, acceptance, and interconnectedness, allowing the melodies of resilience to guide her journey. Her story becomes a part of the symphony of humanity, inspiring us all to embrace our own unique compositions of resilience.

As we reach the final crescendo of "Whispers of Resilience," let us celebrate the symphony of life , the harmonious interplay of our experiences, emotions, and connections. May we conduct our symphonies with courage, grace, and unwavering resilience, knowing that within the symphony lies the power to overcome, to thrive, and to embrace the fullness of our existence.

The symphony continues, and the echoes of resilience resound in every beat of our hearts."

Title%3A %20%22Whispers %20of,of%20our %20hearts.

Printed in Great Britain
by Amazon